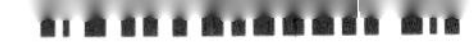

HERBS FOR MALARIA

Unlocking Nature's Healing Power, Harnessing The Therapeutic Potential Of Medicinal Plants

DR. JEREMY ALLEY

Disclaimer:

The information provided in this book, is intended for general informational purposes only and should not be considered as professional advice.

The author has made every effort to ensure the accuracy of the information presented. However, readers are advised to consult with a qualified healthcare professional before attempting any herbal remedies or making significant changes to their wellness routine. Individual health conditions vary, and what may be suitable for one person may not be appropriate for another.

It is important to note that the author is not in any endorsement deal, partnership, or affiliation with any organization, brand, or company mentioned in this book. Any references to specific products or services are based on the author's personal experience or general knowledge and do not imply an endorsement or promotion of those products or services.

Contents

Overview

The Plasmodium parasite is the infectious agent that causes malaria, an illness spread by mosquitoes. It is still a major global health risk, especially in areas that are tropical or subtropical. Herbal treatments have long been used as a management and prevention option for malaria, notwithstanding scientific advances in the field. This article explores the basics of malaria and highlights the use of herbal remedies in treating the disease.

About The Book

Humans can contract malaria from the bites of female Anopheles mosquitoes carrying the potentially fatal virus. Fever, chills, headaches, and muscle aches are among the symptoms; if left untreated, they frequently result in serious consequences. There are multiple species of the parasite Plasmodium, the most deadly of which is P.

falciparum. Low-income nations are disproportionately affected by malaria, which places a significant strain on public health systems.

Even while traditional anti-malarial medications are frequently used for both treatment and prevention, there are still issues with their pricing and accessibility, particularly in environments with limited resources. As a result, there is increasing interest in investigating herbal medicines as adjunctive or alternative methods of treating malaria.

The Value of Herbal Treatments

For generations, herbal treatments have been an integral part of conventional medical systems. Many communities, especially in areas where malaria is widespread, rely on the medicinal qualities of several plants to reduce symptoms and strengthen immunity. The potential of herbal therapies to provide sustainable and affordable solutions makes them significant in the context of malaria.

Sweet Wormwood's (Artemisia annua) artemisinin

Artemisinin, which is extracted from the plant Artemisia annua, popularly known as sweet wormwood, is one of the most well-known herbal treatments for malaria. The World Health Organization (WHO) now generally recommends artemisinin-based combination treatments (ACTs) for the treatment of simple malaria. Due to its quick and strong anti-malarial actions, artemisinin and its derivatives are extremely useful in the fight against the illness.

Bark of Cinchona (Quinine)

There is a long history of using cinchona bark, which contains the alkaloid quinine, to cure malaria. Quinine was a key component in the creation of anti-malarial medications and is still used in certain situations today. It functions by impeding the parasite's capacity to metabolize hemoglobin, which finally causes the parasite to perish. Despite quinine's effectiveness, it's crucial to remember that due to possible side effects, usage should be carefully controlled.

Malaria and Neem (Azadirachta indica)

The Indian subcontinent's natural neem tree has become well-known for its anti-malarial qualities. Neem tree components, including leaves and seeds, have been shown to contain substances that have anti-malarial properties. Neem extracts show promise as a therapy and preventative measure because of their capacity to impede the growth of the malaria parasite.

Wormwood from Africa (Artemisia afra)

A close relative of sweet wormwood, African wormwood has long been used in African herbal medicine to treat malaria. The plant has substances with anti-malarial qualities that are comparable to artemisinin. Although further investigation is required to confirm its effectiveness, African wormwood exhibits potential as a natural treatment for malaria.

When it comes to treating and preventing malaria, herbal medicines are quite important. For people who are unable to obtain traditional therapies, the tremendous biodiversity of plants provides an enormous assortment of chemicals with anti-malarial capabilities. Herbal medicines should be used cautiously, nevertheless, as there is a need for thorough scientific research to confirm their effectiveness and guarantee their safe application in the fight against malaria.

CHAPTER ONE

COMMUNICATION WITH MALARIA

Plasmodium parasites, which cause malaria, are a potentially fatal disease spread by the bites of female Anopheles mosquitoes. It is still a major global health risk, especially in areas that are tropical or subtropical. Comprehending the parasite's life cycle in the human body is essential to understanding the range of therapeutic options available, including herbal therapies.

Reasons And Signs

Five distinct Plasmodium parasite species are the main cause of malaria, with Plasmodium falciparum being the most lethal. Through mosquito bites, the parasites enter the bloodstream and eventually make their way into the liver and red blood cells. Fever, chills, sweats, exhaustion, nausea, and body aches are typical symptoms. Severe consequences from malaria, including organ failure and death, can occur if treatment is not received. It is essential to comprehend these causes and symptoms to act promptly.

Herbal Remedies Vs. Conventional Therapies

Historically, the treatment of malaria in conventional medicine has involved the use of antimalarial medications such as artemisinin-based combination treatments (ACTs) and chloroquine.

Despite the effectiveness of these drugs, worries have been raised by the rise of drug-resistant forms.

On the other hand, herbal therapies have been utilized as supplemental or alternative malaria treatments for ages in a variety of civilizations. The advantages and disadvantages of both herbal remedies and conventional medical treatments can be better understood by contrasting them.

Antiplasmodial herbs are frequently used in herbal therapies for malaria. One well-known example is artemisinin, which is extracted from the sweet wormwood plant (Artemisia annua). Because of its effectiveness, this chemical has been added to various traditional antimalarial medications. Furthermore, quinine-containing Cinchona bark has long been used to treat malaria.

These herbal remedies demonstrate the wide variety of plant-based remedies that have antimalarial qualities.

Many herbs are useful in the treatment of malaria because they naturally have antimalarial qualities. Azadirachta indica, or neem, is known for its anti-inflammatory and antiparasitic qualities.

 Traditional medicine has employed the bark and leaves of the neem tree to treat malaria.

Similarly, an extract from the roots of the West African native plant Cryptolepis sanguinolenta has demonstrated potential in the treatment of malaria. Examining these herbal remedies offers a more comprehensive viewpoint on possible substitutes for traditional medical interventions.

Herbal treatments for malaria present a lot of hope, but there are drawbacks as well, such as inconsistent dosing and possible adverse effects.

Furthermore, research on the scientific validation of these therapies' safety and efficacy is still ongoing. To ensure a more thorough and successful malaria treatment plan, it is imperative to bridge the gap between conventional and herbal therapies by incorporating traditional knowledge with contemporary scientific methodologies.

Developing effective treatments for malaria requires a thorough understanding of the disease's etiology and symptoms.

The contrast between herbal remedies and conventional methods highlights the necessity of treating malaria with a comprehensive and integrated strategy. Investigating herbal therapies indicates a wide range of plants that may have antimalarial qualities, which aids in the continuous fight against this worldwide health issue.

CHAPTER TWO

HERBS TO PREVENT MALARIA

The Plasmodium parasite, which causes malaria, is a mosquito-borne disease that can be fatal. It continues to be a major global health concern. Herbal treatments have drawn interest due to their potential in both controlling and preventing malaria, even if standard antimalarial medications are still commonly utilized for therapy. This section examines several botanicals with anti-malarial qualities.

Sweet Wormwood, Artemisia Annua

Sweet Wormwood, or Artemisia annua, has been a main focus in the hunt for all-natural anti-malaria treatments. Artemisinin is a chemical found in the plant that has strong antimalarial effects. The plant itself has been used for centuries in Chinese medicine, and artemisinin-based combination treatments (ACTs) are commonly utilized in conventional medicine. According to research, Artemisia annua may provide preventive benefits in addition to aiding in the treatment of malaria.

Bark Of Cinchona (Quinine)

There is a long history of using quinine-rich cinchona bark to treat malaria.

One of the first recognized remedies for the illness, quinine, works well against the Plasmodium parasite.

Its natural form found in Cinchona bark is acknowledged for its capacity to prevent malaria, even though it is often found in pharmaceutical antimalarial drugs.

The medicinal benefits of Cinchona bark are frequently linked to its bitter flavor, and herbal cures using the bark may provide an alternate or supplementary method to traditional therapies.

The Azadirachta indica tree yields neem, which is well-known for its many health benefits, including its ability to combat malaria.

The neem tree's leaves, seeds, and bark are among its parts that contain substances with anti-parasitic properties such as reducing and nimbidin. In Ayurvedic medicine, neem has long been used to treat infectious disorders like malaria. The tree may be useful in preventing malaria because of its bitter flavor and immune-system-modulating properties.

Eucalyptus

Notable for its fragrant leaves and oil, eucalyptus is another herbal medicine that has demonstrated potential in combating malaria. Cineole is one of the chemicals found in eucalyptus leaf essential oil, which has anti-inflammatory and antimalarial activities. Although eucalyptus is frequently related to respiratory health, its capacity to repel mosquitoes—who are responsible for spreading the Plasmodium parasite—explains its role in preventing malaria.

Garlic

The possibility of garlic, a culinary herb with well-established therapeutic characteristics, to prevent malaria has also been investigated. Garlic's main ingredient, allicin, has antibacterial qualities and may help explain why the herb is considered anti-malarial. Garlic's use as a natural mosquito repellent and immune system booster implies a potential function in reducing the beginning of malaria, but further research is needed to fully appreciate its efficacy against the disease.

Although there has been interest in using herbal medicines to prevent malaria, it is important to use caution when using them.

To guarantee that herbal therapies are safely and successfully included in current preventative programs, consultation with healthcare professionals is essential, particularly in areas where malaria is endemic. The investigation of these herbs emphasizes how crucial it is to integrate traditional wisdom with cutting-edge science to create all-encompassing strategies in the fight against malaria.

Treatment For Malaria Using Herbal Remedies

The Plasmodium parasite, which causes malaria, is a mosquito-borne disease that can be fatal. Malaria remains a global health concern. Herbal medicines have drawn attention due to their possible therapeutic effects, even if conventional drugs are still commonly employed for therapy. Numerous plants have proven to have anti-malarial qualities, providing supplementary or alternate methods of treating this contagious illness.

Papaya Leaf Extract

One of the most well-known herbal treatments for malaria is papaya leaf extract. According to studies, substances in papaya leaves have anti-malarial properties that prevent the Plasmodium parasite from growing. The extract's anti-malarial properties may be aided by the abundance of enzymes like papain in it. Papaya leaf extract is also well known for its capacity to strengthen the immune system, which helps the body fight off infections more successfully.

Ginger

The anti-malarial properties of ginger, a frequently used spice and medicinal herb, have been investigated. Studies reveal that ginger possesses bioactive substances that have anti-parasitic properties against Plasmodium. Additionally, ginger contains antioxidant and anti-inflammatory qualities that can help reduce malaria symptoms including fever and inflammation. During the treatment of malaria, adding ginger to the diet or drinking ginger tea may offer some alleviation.

Ginger

The Curcuma longa plant yields turmeric, a bright yellow spice that is well-known for its anti-inflammatory and antioxidant qualities. The key ingredient in turmeric, curcumin, has been researched for possible anti-malarial properties. Early on in an infection, curcumin may prevent the Plasmodium parasite from developing, according to research. Adding turmeric to one's diet or supplementing with it could help manage the symptoms of malaria overall.

The King of Bitters, Andrographis paniculata

The herb Andrographis paniculata, also referred to as the King of Bitters, has long been used in traditional medicine to treat a variety of illnesses, including malaria. The active ingredients in Andrographis paniculata, andrographolides, have been shown in studies to have anti-malarial qualities. These substances have the potential to alter the immune response and stop the Plasmodium parasite from growing. This herb's extracts can be found in a variety of formats, including tinctures and capsules, which makes them accessible to people looking for alternative treatments for malaria.

Extract From Olive Leaf

Olive leaf extract, which has antibacterial qualities, is made from the leaves of the olive tree (Olea europaea).

According to research, olive leaf extract may inhibit the Plasmodium parasite's life cycle, which would provide anti-malarial properties. Furthermore, the extract has substances that have anti-inflammatory and antioxidant qualities, which may help lessen malaria symptoms.

Olive leaf extract is a practical alternative for anyone looking for herbal therapies for malaria, as it comes in a variety of forms, such as capsules and liquid extracts.

Although they won't replace traditional medical care, herbal remedies for malaria may offer additional support and help with symptom relief. Especially in areas where malaria is common, it is imperative to speak with medical professionals before adding herbal treatments to the treatment regimen. Herbal therapies have differing degrees of effectiveness and individual responses, which highlights the need for individualized healthcare in the treatment of this infectious condition.

CHAPTER THREE

HERBAL SOLUTIONS FOR MACROPHAGE

The infectious disease malaria, which is spread by mosquitoes and is brought on by Plasmodium parasites, is still a major threat to world health. Even while there are conventional medical treatments available, some people look for alternative methods to promote their recovery and reduce symptoms, like herbal medicines. We investigate the use of herbal infusions, teas, tinctures, and pills as possible treatments for malaria in this investigation.

Formulas And Combinations Of Herbs

A comprehensive strategy for treating malaria symptoms is provided by herbal formulae and combinations. Certain herbal mixtures are used in traditional medical systems, like Ayurveda and traditional Chinese medicine, to treat the infection.

Neem, Cinchona bark, and Artemisia annua (sweet wormwood) are among the ingredients whose anti-malarial qualities have been acknowledged. It's commonly believed that these mixtures increase the treatment's overall effectiveness by acting in concert.

Herbal remedies can also be customized to a person's constitution and the particular malaria parasite strain that affects them. Although the process of scientific validation for these formulations is still ongoing, historical usage and anecdotal evidence point to the potential benefits of herbal combinations as valuable adjuncts to malaria management measures.

Herbal Teas

For many years, people have drank herbal teas for their medicinal qualities, and some herbs are thought to contain anti-malarial capabilities. Sweet wormwood, or Artemisia annua, is a prominent element in a lot of herbal teas that fight malaria. Artemisinin, a substance known for its strong anti-malarial effects, is found in the plant.

Because of their ability to strengthen the immune system and reduce inflammation, additional herbs like ginger, cinnamon, and cloves are frequently added to these teas. Herbal teas can help reduce symptoms and promote general well-being during the healing process for malaria, even if they might not be a stand-alone treatment. But, it's important to speak with medical experts before depending just on herbal drinks to treat malaria.

Extracts And Tinctures

The convenient and effective administration of therapeutic plants is made possible by the concentrated forms of plants found in herbal tinctures and extracts. Herbs including Artemisia annua, Cinchona bark, and Cryptolepis sanguinolenta can be used to make tinctures for malaria. It is thought that these extracts, which are frequently used orally, affect the malaria parasite by interfering with its life cycle.

Tinctures have the benefit of being rapidly absorbed, which may accelerate the beginning of therapeutic benefits.

 However, as incorrect use may result in negative consequences or diminished efficacy, the dosage and formulation of herbal tinctures should be carefully evaluated.

To guarantee safe and efficient use, like with any alternative treatment, speaking with healthcare professionals is crucial.

Herbal Supplements

Herbal capsules offer encapsulated herbal treatments in a handy form, facilitating accurate dosage. Like herbal teas and tinctures, anti-malarial plants like neem and Artemisia annua are frequently included in capsule form. For those who may not find herbal teas appealing, the encapsulating procedure might help hide the occasionally bitter flavor of certain plants, making them more pleasant.

However, several variables, including the quality of the herbs utilized, the method of extraction, and individual response variability, affect how effective herbal capsules are.

To guarantee correct dosage and avoid any possible drug interactions, caution must be used. It is advisable to incorporate herbal capsules into malaria management under the supervision of medical professionals.

there are many different ways that herbal treatments for malaria can be used, including properly mixed mixtures, teas, tinctures, and capsules.

Traditional medicine and anecdotal reports acknowledge the potential benefits of these treatments; however, to achieve comprehensive malaria management, it is crucial to approach these remedies with a balanced perspective, integrating traditional knowledge with scientific evidence and consulting healthcare professionals.

CHAPTER FOUR

HYPOTENSIVE SUPPORT FOR THE RECOVERY OF MALARIA

Plasmodium parasites are the cause of malaria, an infectious disease spread by mosquitoes that continues to be a danger to world health. Herbal therapies and nutritional assistance can be beneficial in the healing process, even while traditional medical treatments like antimalarial drugs are essential for controlling the illness. This article explores the value of supplements, suggested diets, and nutrition in helping those afflicted with malaria.

Nutrition's Significance

In addition to being vital for general health, adequate nutrition is even more important during and after a malaria infection. Malaria can cause several side effects, such as reduced immunity and anemia. Sufficient nourishment can boost the immune system, assist the body to recuperate, and restore the body's energy reserves. Vital nutrients from a diet that is well-balanced aid in the recovery of health and vigor.

Malnutrition can worsen the symptoms of malaria and lengthen the time it takes to recover. Severe malaria may be more likely to strike people with weakened immune systems or undernourished bodies. As a result, giving nutritional support top priority is crucial for controlling and mitigating the symptoms of this viral disease.

Suggested Nutrition

A nutritious, well-balanced diet is essential for those recuperating from malaria. The immune system can be strengthened and depleted nutrients can be replenished by emphasizing foods high in vitamins, minerals, and antioxidants. Dietary staples should include nutritious grains, lean proteins, fresh produce, and healthy fats.

More specifically, anemia—a typical side effect of malaria—can be treated with meals strong in iron, such as leafy green vegetables, lean meats, and legumes. Citrus fruits and other foods high in vitamin C improve the absorption of iron from plant-based sources. Including zinc-rich foods like nuts, seeds, and whole grains can also boost the immune system and speed up the healing process.

Another essential component of the diet that is suggested for recovering from malaria is hydration. Malaria's fever and perspiration can cause dehydration, so it's critical to drink plenty of water, herbal teas, and electrolyte-rich liquids.

Addenda

Although eating whole foods is the best way to get nutrients, supplements can also be helpful, particularly in cases of severe malnutrition or trouble sticking to a varied diet. Supplements containing many vitamins and minerals can offer a wide variety of nutrients to support general health as the body heals.

Furthermore, depending on a person's requirements and deficits, some supplements like zinc, vitamin C, and iron may be taken into consideration.

Supplemental herbal remedies also aid in the recovery from malaria.

Research on the antimalarial effects of artemisinin, which is extracted from the sweet wormwood plant (Artemisia annua), has been conducted.

But before using herbal supplements, it's important to speak with a doctor because certain herbal supplements have contraindications for particular illnesses or may conflict with drugs.

A crucial part of the all-encompassing strategy for treating malaria is nutritional assistance.

A balanced diet that is high in vital nutrients can help those who are afflicted with this infectious condition heal more quickly, experience fewer symptoms, and feel better overall. To prevent malaria and promote long-term health, a complete and effective strategy combining dietary assistance with traditional medical treatments is necessary.

CHAPTER FIVE

SAFETY OF HERBAL MEDICINE AND PRECAUTIONS

For millennia, people have used herbal treatments as a natural substitute for pharmaceuticals while treating malaria.

Even though these treatments have some efficacy, it is important to put safety first and understand any potential risks before using them.

People should speak with medical specialists before adding herbal remedies to a malaria treatment plan, especially in areas where the disease is common.

It is crucial to understand that, despite their potential benefits, herbal therapies cannot replace prescription antimalarial drugs.

Guidelines For Dosage

It's critical to establish the right dosage for herbal treatments to maximize their effectiveness and reduce the possibility of side effects.

The exact herbal medicine being used, the severity of the malaria infection, and individual factors like age, weight, and general health may all affect the dosage recommendations.

To create a precise and unique dosage regimen, speaking with a licensed herbalist or healthcare professional is crucial.

It is best to begin with a smaller dosage and increase it gradually while keeping an eye out for any negative reactions or evidence of improvement.

Potential Relationships

Malaria herbal medicines may interact with other drugs or substances, which could reduce their effectiveness or have unfavorable effects.

It is important to be aware of potential interactions between conventional antimalarial treatments and herbal remedies, as well as other medications a person may be taking for unrelated ailments.

All substances used, including herbal supplements, should be disclosed to healthcare practitioners so they can evaluate any possible interactions and modify treatment regimens as necessary.

The field of herb-drug interactions is always changing, therefore it's critical to stay up to date on the most recent discoveries.

Restrictions

Due to contraindications, certain people may need to proceed with caution or stay away from certain herbal medicines completely.

These disqualifications may be caused by pregnancy, underlying medical disorders, or other conditions that raise the possibility of negative side effects. For example, people who are allergic to specific plants, have liver problems or are pregnant may not be able to use some herbs.

To avoid complications and guarantee the safety of herbal treatments in the treatment of malaria, a thorough grasp of contraindications is essential.

When it's essential, healthcare professionals can evaluate each patient's health profile to find any contraindications and suggest alternate treatments.

Although they can make a significant therapeutic contribution, herbal medicines for malaria must be used with caution, taking into account personal health histories and safety concerns.

The use of herbal medication in a comprehensive treatment plan for malaria necessitates adherence to dosage standards, knowledge of potential interactions, and comprehension of contraindications.

People can maximize the advantages of these all-natural options while lowering the hazards by using herbal therapies with caution and knowledge.

CHAPTER SIX

CASE RESEARCH

Case studies provide a thorough analysis of specific experiences of herbal medicines for malaria in individuals. These studies, which record the results and effects on the patients, frequently entail the usage of particular herbs or herbal formulations. Using artemisinin, a natural extract made from the sweet wormwood plant, is one noteworthy case study. The study investigates the potential benefits of artemisinin-based combination therapies (ACTs) over traditional antimalarial medications as well as their efficacy in treating malaria.

A further case study might concentrate on the customary application of herbal remedies in particular areas, illustrating how local populations have incorporated plant-based therapies into their medical practices. These examples provide light on the variety of herbal remedies and the range of success rates for them.

Achievement Stories

Success tales describe cases where people have used herbal treatments to successfully treat malaria. These narratives frequently highlight the successful outcomes and enhanced health of individuals who have used herbal remedies in conjunction with conventional malaria treatment. The usage of quinine, which is made from the bark of the cinchona tree, as a historically significant and successful herbal treatment for treating malaria is one such success story.

Examining the success stories of people who have mixed herbal medicines with medical therapies can help reveal possible areas of overlap between various therapeutic modalities. These accounts add to the increasing amount of data that supports the use of herbal medications in malaria treatment regimens.

Actual Occurrences

Experiences from everyday life offer a more comprehensive viewpoint on the usefulness of herbal treatments for malaria. Testimonials from people who have chosen herbal therapies could be included in this part, describing their experiences, difficulties they have encountered, and general happiness with the results. The aforementioned anecdotes enhance our comprehension of the intricate process of integrating herbal treatments into the treatment of malaria.

Furthermore, real-world encounters could explore the cultural facets of herbal therapy and how cultures with a strong herbal knowledge base cure malaria. Discussions about the cultural importance of herbal treatments and their use in public health policies can benefit from insights gained from these experiences.

Herbal treatments for malaria provide a complex and dynamic method of managing the illness. Real-world experiences, case studies, and success stories all add to the expanding body of research demonstrating the possible effectiveness of herbal remedies.

While appreciating the value of traditional medicine, learning about and comprehending the various applications of herbal medicines offers insightful information for medical professionals and anyone looking for all-encompassing methods of treating and preventing malaria.

CHAPTER SEVEN

HERBALISM AND CLASSICAL MEDICATION METHODS

For ages, the use of herbs, a practice with strong roots in traditional healing techniques, has played a major role in healthcare across many countries. Herbal treatments have been quite helpful in the context of malaria in terms of relieving and supporting those afflicted with this potentially fatal illness. The historical significance and current applicability of herbalism in the treatment of malaria are examined in this section.

The Function Of Conventional Medicine

Herbal medicines, which are part of traditional medicine, have historically been essential in treating health issues such as malaria.

Indigenous groups all around the world have amassed a vast collection of therapeutic herbs that are effective against the malaria parasite. Comprehending the function of traditional medicine about malaria illuminates the significant contributions that herbal treatments make to the field of global health.

Herbal knowledge that has been passed down through the decades has been guarded by traditional healers, who are frequently highly embedded in their communities.

Their proficiency in recognizing and employing therapeutic herbs has been important in combating malaria.

Healthcare systems can investigate synergies that close the gap between conventional and herbal therapies by acknowledging the significance of traditional medicine.

This will ultimately improve the overall efficacy of malaria treatment and prevention strategies.

Herbal medicine's incorporation into traditional healthcare systems is a viable approach to tackling the intricate problems caused by malaria. In addition to providing an extra layer of support and possibly reducing problems like drug resistance, traditional herbal medicines can be used in conjunction with mainstream antimalarial medications.

The many ways that herbalism can be subtly incorporated into medical procedures to improve the overall treatment of malaria are covered in this section.

Promoting cooperation between conventional healers and contemporary medical professionals is one facet of integration.

The two mindsets can be bridged by establishing forums for respectful communication and knowledge sharing.

This cooperative endeavor may result in the discovery of effective herbal treatments, their scientific confirmation, and their integration into conventional medical practices.

Herbal medicine can also be incorporated into healthcare through research and development projects that investigate the therapeutic potential of medicinal plants.

Extensive scientific research on the effectiveness, safety, and dose of herbal therapies can offer the proof required to justify their inclusion in recommended treatments for malaria.

This evidence-based strategy guarantees that herbal medicine develops into a respectable and trustworthy part of medical procedures.

To optimize the management of malaria, it is imperative to acknowledge the historical significance of herbalism, comprehend the function of traditional medicine, and actively work towards the integration of herbal therapies into mainstream healthcare.

In the continuous fight against malaria, society can create a holistic strategy that combines the benefits of modern medicine and herbalism by embracing the wealth of information inherent in traditional healing traditions.

CHAPTER EIGHT

GARDENING WITH HERBS FOR MALARIA REMEDIES

Malaria, a potentially fatal illness spread by parasites that are contracted by mosquito bites, is still a major global health issue.

Herbal treatments provide an alternate method of treating malaria, even if traditional therapy is still quite important.

A sustainable supply of medicinal plants can be obtained by creating an herbal garden specifically designed to treat malaria.

The process of designing such a garden is examined in this guide, from choosing and cultivating medicinal herbs to gathering and preserving them for maximum benefit.

Choosing And Planting Therapeutic Herbs

A successful herbal garden for the treatment of malaria must have the correct herbs. Sweet wormwood, or Artemisia annua, is a strong herb having anti-malarial qualities.

Sunlight and well-drained soil are necessary for its cultivation. Azadirachta indica, or neem, is another priceless botanical with anti-parasitic qualities. Neem trees are appropriate for malaria-affected areas since they grow well in tropical and subtropical climates.

Other plants including Cinchona (Cinchona officinalis), Andrographis (Andrographis paniculata), and Eucalyptus (Eucalyptus globulus) can be taken into consideration in addition to Artemisia annua and Neem.

A successful herbal garden necessitates an understanding of the particular growing conditions, soil requirements, and climate preferences of each herb. The health and efficacy of medicinal plants are influenced by proper spacing, irrigation, and gardening practices.

Gathering And Preserving Herbs

The therapeutic effectiveness of herbs is greatly influenced by the time of harvest. The optimal time to harvest plants is when their concentration of active chemicals is at its peak.

The blossoming stage of Artemisia annua is frequently regarded as ideal.

Usually, neem leaves are collected before the tree blossoms. Mature trees provide the best sources of quinine, especially in the form of cinchona bark.

After harvesting, the herbs must be properly dried and stored to retain their effectiveness. Herbs' essential oils and active ingredients can be preserved by drying them in a well-ventilated, shady location. Avoiding direct sunlight exposure is crucial since it might cause the quality of medicines to deteriorate.

To keep light and moisture from compromising the quality of the herbs, store them in sealed containers in a cool, dark place after they have dried.

Creating an herbal garden to treat malaria demands dedication to environmentally friendly methods. In addition to traditional malaria treatment, people and communities can obtain a natural and sustainable source of cures by carefully choosing, cultivating, harvesting, and conserving therapeutic herbs.

In addition to improving health, this all-encompassing strategy encourages the growth of beneficial plants that can aid the larger community in the fight against malaria.

FINAL VERDICT

For a considerable amount of time, malaria has been treated with herbal therapies. Traditional medical systems have acknowledged the antimalarial qualities of herbs such as sweet wormwood, cinchona bark, neem, African wormwood, and feverfew. While some herbal remedies are already part of conventional medicine, others are still being studied.

Herbal therapies should be used carefully, taking into account things like dose, possible adverse effects, and combinations with prescription antimalarial medications. As this field of study progresses, herbal remedies might provide further assistance in the global fight against malaria.

Recap Of Herbal Remedies

A review of many herbal treatments with possible antimalarial effects was given in this article. Due to its high artemisinin content, sweet wormwood is now a major component of contemporary antimalarial therapies. Neem, African Wormwood, Feverfew, and Cinchona Bark all show the potential to reduce malaria symptoms. Although there are alternatives provided by traditional herbal treatments, it is important to recognize that further research is necessary to confirm their safety and efficacy.

A holistic strategy that combines conventional and herbal therapies may offer a more effective approach to the treatment and prevention of malaria as the world struggles with its problems.

www.ingramcontent.com/pod-product-compliance
Lightning Source LLC
Chambersburg PA
CBHW060842260726
48661CB00002B/561